Wounded:

My Battle to Overcome Anxiety and Depression

N. Montour

WOUNDED:

My Battle to Overcome
Anxiety and Depression

If you are in danger of hurting yourself,
please call the
National Suicide Prevention Hotline
at
(800) 273-8255

Contents

Introduction

Chapter 1 The Slow Decent into Darkness: A Brief History

Chapter 2 Trying to See in The Dark – Living with Anxiety and Depression

Chapter 3 The Journey of Discovery – Finding Solutions to Overcome Anxiety and Depression

Chapter 4 The Results – What I Found Most Helpful

Chapter 5 The Future

INTRODUCTION

"Promise me you'll always remember that you're braver than you believe, stronger than you seem, and smarter than you think." Christopher Robin to Winnie the Pooh. Thank you for purchasing this book. I want to begin by saying by no means do I want you to think I am an expert in the topic of anxiety and depression, but I have personally experienced and lived it. I know what it feels like, and I understand the deep dark struggles that millions of people are going through each day. Thoughts and emotions are powerful things, as I'm sure you know. According to the World Health Organization, "Globally, more than 300 million people suffer from depression, and 260 million suffer from anxiety disorders—many of whom live with both conditions." Honestly, I wonder how accurate those numbers are. I truly believe that everyone in this world either lives with or knows someone who is dealing with anxiety and/or depression, even if they are not aware of it. Remarkably, many people interact with people they don't even know are experiencing anxiety and/or depression. It is such a terrible affliction that I can easily say that I could never wish the torture associated with mental illness on my worst enemy. For those who do not experience or have not experienced the pains associated with anxiety and depression, it can be very difficult to relate to or even empathize with those who do or have. What is hard for one person may not be hard for others, but each of us has our own challenges and struggles in life, and I think it's important to help anyone struggling to find peace and recognize the joys and beauty of life. I know how hard it is, but it's possible. My whole life, I have suffered alone and wished I could reach out or find someone to help me through it all.

My goal for this book is to help those who suffer in silence and offer hope and guidance to live life happier and find a little peace and contentment. Every day, I see news stories about suicide and misery around the world, and it hurts to think how many people are suffering. I have been looking for ways to reach out and help as many people as I can. I think it is so vital that everyone knows they are not alone. After many attempts, I decided this book might be the best way to reach a larger audience. Since those who experience anxiety and depression often find it hard to get out and interact with people, and even share their darkest fears and worries, I hope this book will afford many the opportunity to look deeper within themselves and find solutions when the time is right.

Since you are reading this, I expect you want help and answers. So, I have tried to keep this book short, easy to read and to the point. I will walk you through a little of my life that may have led to the despair and struggles I have experienced. Then I will summarize my path to find solutions for overcoming anxiety and depression and where each solution led me. My goal is to try and help you see that there is always hope, no matter how bad things may look. I sincerely hope this book will help you or someone you know find the help to finally overcome the struggles of anxiety and depression.

"I don't know where my story will end,

but nowhere will it read ...

I gave up!"

CHAPTER 1

The Slow Decent into Darkness: A Brief History

I don't want to bore you with a long, drawn-out story of my life. I just want to give you a little background as to who I am and where I came from so you can better see what led to my issues with anxiety and depression. Hopefully you can relate and see that there is hope for a better life

I was born in Canada; my mother was American, and my father was Canadian. My father had a tough life growing up, having been kicked out of the house at 13 years of age because he was the oldest of 10 and his parents decided he was one more mouth they couldn't feed. Despite his difficult childhood, he survived and became an uneducated engineer, learning from friends who helped him along. Luckily, he was able to take advantage of on-the-job training in the oil industry, which gave him a career path. However, being uneducated meant he couldn't find permanent employment without being paid very little, so he took what he could get through contract work. As a result of this career instability, we moved a lot. We had to go wherever and for however long the contract work happened to be. We seemed to be on the move every six months to a year, from one place to another throughout the United States and Canada. All this moving and looking for work also meant money was tight. So, we had very little in terms of material things and no stability in our lives.

I am the second youngest of five kids, so I was like a middle child. I felt hated my whole life growing up. Whether or not that was true, I really have no idea, but if you go through life believing that, it becomes true, at least to you. I was closest to my younger brother, who I dragged around with me on whatever adventure I could find. I have always been a very independent person, even at a young age. I recognized early on that my parents didn't have money, so I decided if I wanted to buy or do anything, I would have to take responsibility to do it myself. So, at the age of 10, I got a paper route. Let me tell you, it is hard enough getting up so early in the morning, but it was even harder during the cold Canadian winters. The money I made brought me some freedom, even if it just meant being able to go to the gas station to buy myself a box of small powdered donuts, which I still love to this day. I delivered papers until I turned 15, at which age I could finally get a "real" job. I got hired at the greatest place in the world for a 15-year old who loved to eat: McDonald's. I loved McDonald's. I will never forget my first day, when the manager asked if I enjoyed eating the food there, and I promptly told him yes to which he replied, "Not for much longer. You will get sick of it." Well, I proved him wrong. My younger brother and I would have contests to see who could eat more Big Macs, and life was good! I worked the grill, and it was exciting getting the burgers out to hungry customers as quickly as I could cook and build them. In my young 15-year-old mind, it seemed like I was making thousands of burgers each day. Closing shift was a sad time for me, because it meant all the food that didn't sell would be thrown away. I wanted more than anything to take it home and eat it, but the manager would never allow it. It was such a waste.

I loved what my work experience did for me when I was younger. I brought me freedom to do what I wanted to do, which was primarily buying food and going to the local arcade to drop as many quarters as I could in the latest games. But the biggest challenge I faced growing up was all the moving. We were always the new kids, and it sucked. Kids can be cruel, as I'm sure most of you would agree. One advantage I had was that I was a big kid.

Not fat, but tall. Yet this still didn't stop other kids from ganging up on me. They all wanted to be the ones who took down the new big kid. I suppose I am proud to say I have never lost a fight, even when it was four or five to one. I only started one fight with a kid who wouldn't stop making fun of me, and I figured it was the only way to shut him up. Well, I beat him up, and he stopped making fun of me, but I didn't feel better. I felt bad about making him fight. But it made me feel worse watching him walk away with all his friends while I walked home all alone. Moving around all the time was hard, acceptable, or cool ways to talk or do things in one place was not necessarily cool in another. I got so tired of being the target of jokes and made fun of day after day. All this forced me to become an introvert and super shy, just keeping to myself in order to avoid drama. This is ironic because I love being around people and having fun, but when you don't have friends, what choice do you have? I became the silent observer. It got to the point where I was afraid to say anything to anyone. It was so bad, I would barely say more than two words even to my parents. I was afraid to say express myself or do anything in front of anyone for fear of being made fun of. I hated it. I also thought of myself as the black sheep of my family. I was that classic middle child who felt like everyone hated him. I felt excluded and so very alone. All this led down a path to depression and anxiety that would impact me for years to come.

One major difference I noticed among the kids at school was the stability they all seemed to have, including extended family. I was jealous hearing about other kids going away on vacations, and having family reunions, and seeing their cousins and uncles and aunts and grandparents. It sounded so wonderful. I would dream of having family like that one day. But I didn't have much hope, since not even my own brothers and sister liked me.

When I was a junior in high school, we moved to Tacoma, Washington, and I started at yet another new school, Curtis High School. There, I became an A/V geek. I also did theater production and really enjoyed set building, lighting, and all the technical aspects of making a play come to life. I had participated in a few sports, but my only advantage was my size. I was six feet eight inches tall by the time I was 16, so I easily made the teams. However, I found that, even in high school, the politics in sports were more than I wanted to deal with, so by senior year I quit sports. I took a lot of trade classes like auto repair, wood and metal working, and welding. I am good with my hands and loved to take things apart just to see how they worked. As I kid, I was always finding old radios and stuff I would fix up and use for years.

At age 17, I knew if I wanted my driver's license, I would have to get it myself. So, thanks to my job working at an ice cream shop, I paid to take a driving course and get my license. A short time later, I knew of a guy whose parents bought him a fancy 1979 Ford Pinto that was bright orange. He hated it and never drove it once, so I offered to buy it from him for $500, and he quickly agreed. I had my first car and it was beautiful! I loved it. This gave me even more independence. My father was quite surprised to find out I not only got my license on my own, but that I bought myself a car, too. His response was basically, "Hmm", whatever that meant. I took it as he was proud of me. Since we never had any money, my dad was always working on our cars. I learned a lot about car repair from him and still love to work on cars today.

I finally made it through high school and got a job working for a cabinet company. We made custom cabinets for homes, shops, or whatever. The job I was tasked with when not helping with cabinets was making audio cassette tape and CD racks. It felt like I made a million of them. I would build these racks for 8 hours a day.

By this time, my dad had found work in a small town called Ponca City, Oklahoma. He and my mom moved down there so they could find a place to live and get set up, allowing us kids to stay behind until my youngest brother finished high school. A lot happened during that time. My father was diagnosed with cancer and needed urgent surgery to remove his kidney and the cancer. I was working two jobs to help pay the bills. I built cabinets by day and cleaned restaurants by night. The highlight of the night was meeting up with my oldest brother at the restaurant he worked at and watching David Letterman on the bar's big screen TV while eating popcorn.

Eventually, it was time to move to Oklahoma. At 19 years old, I drove our 26-foot truck from Tacoma, Washington, all the way down to Ponca City, Oklahoma, in about three days. It was a fun trip. I always loved road trips, which is funny because I always get car sick -- but not as a driver. Our go-to music was always Neil Diamond's song, "America". Yes, even though we were from Canada, we loved that song. We got settled in Oklahoma, but it was a small, depressing town. I decided to serve a mission for my church, hoping it would take me somewhere I could learn a new language.

After about three weeks in Ponca City, I left and headed to Recife, Brazil, to start my mission. My first challenge was to learn Portuguese. Despite spending two months at the training center studying the language, I didn't understand anything. Landing in Brazil was scary at first, because I didn't know anything about the country, culture, people, or language. My first night there, the president was impeached and there were demonstrations and rioting in the streets. Not knowing what was going on was frightening. But I carried on, and eventually I picked up the language and loved the people. It really is amazing to learn a new language. It's funny, but I never really noticed I was doing well with my Portuguese until one day it just become natural.

I started out in the main city of Recife, which I didn't like too much. I think it was mainly because I didn't like working with the other Americans. I found them rude, arrogant, and just irritating. After about six months, I moved to the interior of the country and got my wish to be surrounded by just Brazilians. I loved them. Brazilians are just the most wonderful, warmest people in the world. They welcomed me with open arms, and for the first time in my life I felt accepted. It was paradise for me. I loved serving the people and working together and having fun. It was the most incredible time of my life. This is where I learned who God was. God is the smile of every child and the hug of every caring person. God is about serving and loving one another. I found peace. I found relief from the pain of depression and anxiety I had been experiencing for so many years. I would find out later that I would meet my future wife in Brazil. I never wanted it to end.

But unfortunately, all good things must come to an end. After two years I headed home to Oklahoma. As I got off the little prop plane at the tiny Ponca City airport, I found my parents waiting for me, and my father hugged me for the first time I could remember. I was shocked to see how he received me, because I always felt like the unwanted child. It was a nice homecoming, but I was already feeling alone. I came home to an empty house. My brothers and sister were gone, so it was just me and my ailing parents. I came home to a place I never got to know because I was there for only three weeks before I left on the mission. During my time in Brazil, my mother developed a heart problem. IN addition to suffering with that ailment, my father's health never recovered after his cancer surgery. I immediately sought to find work and got a job at the local restaurant as a waiter. I enjoyed it, but, wow, are people cheap! During this time, I was corresponding with my future wife in Brazil. I was planning to head back down to Brazil, and perhaps move there permanently.

About a month after I got back, my dad went back to the doctor and found out the cancer was not only back, but back with a vengeance. It had hold of his other kidney and had spread to his liver and all over his abdomen. The doctor gave him 60 days to live. He was spot on. At just about 60 days later, my father went to bed and never woke up. I was so sad. I finally had the relationship I always dreamed of having with my father, and he died. But I was grateful for what little time I had with him. My two oldest brothers came for the funeral, and it was nice. They left a short time later and I continued to work and carry on as best I could.

I kept saving money for my trip to Brazil, but I also wanted to bring my future wife up to meet my mom. I decided the best way to move things along would be to apply for a fiancé visa so we could get married in both countries. I was told getting that visa would take anywhere from 9 months to a year, just to get a response from immigration, which would be plenty of time to save money and travel down and do a lot of things. However, one week after I sent in my application, I was holding the visa in my hand, and I was told that she had 90 days to enter the country and get married. I was not ready for this. I was shocked. I called her and told her, and she agreed to come. I scrambled to get enough money to buy her a plane ticket and did my best to arrange for everything. It was just insane how quickly everything happened. It didn't even give us any time to think, but maybe that was a good thing. She flew up, and five days later we got married. Crazy, I know, but it felt like it was meant to be. I loved her and she meant the world to me as she stills does. We will be married 25 years this year and she has been my rock and my greatest support. I honestly don't know where I would be without her.

All this craziness meant there was no plan for the future. I had no idea what I was going to do or how I was going to provide for my new family. My new wife struggled with the language, life in this foreign country, and of course leaving her family so far away. Back then it was very hard to communicate due to the expense and availability of telephones to her family. But she trusted me to take care of her and I did my best. We were best friends and spent every moment together. Soon after I got a lead on a job at a major supermarket chain distribution warehouse in the area, and I was told it would be a guaranteed temp-to-hire job. Well, month after month passed, and no job offer came. This meant they could work me to death with no benefits and no opportunity to make any real money. I got tired of it and left to try to find whatever else I could. I got a job at the local gas station selling a lot of gas, cheap cigarettes, and beer. I really wanted to go to college, but I had always been told that if you didn't have money, you couldn't go to college. I decided to learn a trade instead. I looked at the local trade school, found classes for Emergency Medical Technicians (EMTs), and went to school at night. I enjoyed the schooling and thought it would be cool to work as an EMT and then maybe a paramedic. I finished my EMT training and looked for work, but how many EMT jobs were there in a tiny little town? Exactly zero. I got a tip that there were opportunities for EMTs in another state, so we took a chance and moved. Unluckily for me, they didn't accept my schooling, so I was out of work.

It took me a lot longer than I would have liked to find a job, but I finally found one as a delivery driver for an electrical distributor. However, I never in fact drove a truck or made a single delivery. After I had been working in the warehouse for about a month, they offered me a job at the sales counter. That was exciting and I really enjoyed it. My two co-workers had been there for many years, and they were mean and quick to scowl at people. But I really enjoyed learning and interacting with customers, and after a few more months I was offered a position in the office as the inside salesman for the "large job" desk. It was another exciting opportunity to learn and grow. Because they kept promoting me so quickly, though, they didn't actually have to offer me a raise. So, I was still making the same hourly wage as I was hired for as a truck driver. They were taking advantage of me. This was tough because we had a son on the way. That was exciting, but I needed to make more money. Not only was money tight, but my wife was health having issues which would mean all three of her pregnancies would be high risk. So, if you can imagine, that just added to the already building anxiety I was dealing with. During this time my first son was born but unfortunately my wife had to have an emergency c-section which caused me a great deal of anxiety. The doctor said I could lose her and the baby if things don't go well. That was a tough day for me. Due to my wife's health, I was afraid to leave her for fear that I would lose her. Luckily, she was ok and so was my son. But I hate to admit, I had a hard time connecting with my son. I never had a relationship with my father, so I just didn't know how to be a good father to him. I am not going to make excuses, but I failed miserably, and I know I was never there for him the way I should have been while he was growing up. Sure, I was there physically, but not emotionally. I just couldn't get past my own emotional and mental health challenges to be there for him and it makes me sad to think about it.

After a year doing excellent work at my job and receiving several recognitions and awards, I decided I should approach my boss and ask for a raise. He promptly refused. I took a gamble and said if all you are going to pay me is a truck driver's salary, then put me back in the warehouse. He called my bluff and I found myself back in the warehouse. That hit me hard and really destroyed what little self-worth I had. It was a depressing time, and I struggled a great deal with anxiety.

About a month later, I got a couple offers from some of the contractors I was working with, and they offered me a nice raise and opportunity. Things seemed to be looking up. I took a warehouse manager job; it was a great job, and I loved it. I oversaw purchasing and delivery of parts and equipment. I worked under the owner, and he was a great guy, but he decided to retire shortly after I was hired, and my position was eliminated. Lucky me. Another blow to my mental health, as I found myself looking for another job. I found one a little later, but it was not a good move. They promised me a raise and other things, but they never came through on any of them. They lied about everything. I was only there a few months before that job was over. It was hard to deal with the fact that I was unemployed for many months after that, during this time feeling even more dejected and panicked not knowing if or when I would find work.

During this time, I found out there were financial aid opportunities to go to college. The very next day I was at the local university talking with the financial aid office and enrolling in classes. I was finally a college student with hope for the future. During this time, we had another child. The daughter I always wanted. I had seen how beautiful the relationship can be between a father and his daughter and I dreamed of that myself. She was so beautiful, I would spend hours talking to her and even though it was a hard time to have another child when you are unemployed, she brought me peace when I spent time with her. I was so happy that my wife survived another delivery which almost put me over the edge. I seriously don't think I could handle it if I had lost her. My wife dreamed of a large family, but all that did was worry me.

Eventually I found another job with an electrical contractor that was getting a lot of government contracts. It seemed like a good job, but the hours were crazy, and I kept missing class. The owners had substance abuse issues and were getting divorced. One owner would show up drunk or high and expect one of the employees to chauffeur him around all day. He was abusive and mean, which tore the business apart. We didn't know if we would get paid one week to the next, and I watched as the best employees walked out one after another. Eventually it got to the point where I couldn't stay any longer, and I had to walk away. I was sure I could find something else, but it took me nine months to find another job. It was a good job working for a good man who was building a new company. Yet, as much as I was happy to find another job, it just didn't pay enough to cover the bills. I was depressed and desperate and didn't know what to do. I loved my latest boss and was grateful to have *something*, but we were struggling to get by. The past five years had been one depressing disappointment after another. I was losing hope for a better future and life. My anxiety was getting worse.

Then, out of the blue, I got a call about a job opportunity I had thought was dead almost a year earlier. It came with an opportunity to relocate to California. I didn't have to think about it; I immediately said yes. My new boss asked how long I needed to get moved, and I told her two weeks. She was floored that I could be there that quickly. I immediately went into my boss's office and gave him my two weeks' notice, and then I went home and told my wife. She wasn't so sure it would work out, but what other option did we have? We had to take a chance. We drove down to Southern California and found our new home. It was so exciting to be living in California. Things finally seemed like they were working out for us. I didn't want to depend only on my new job, so I got enrolled in school to get my degree. I continued to work full time and go to school. Life was hard, but we could pay the bills and there was hope for the future now that I was enrolled in school. Yet, as you can imagine, working full time, going to school, and having a family is very stressful and hard to balance, but I managed. After a few years, I got a transfer to a little farther north, for more money and a better opportunity, and we were there for eight years. That was longer than I had ever lived anywhere in my life. Our last son was born during this time which was a miracle due to my wife's health problems. But she and the baby were fine. For the first time in my life, things seemed to be going ok. I had friends and we were happy. Life was better than I had ever experienced till then.

In 2011, we took a vacation to Brazil to visit my wife's family. It was a nice trip, but I had to come home early for work, and that is when life took a turn for the worse. My boss didn't have much experience in my management area, and she felt like she was in my shadow. She had been passed up for a promotion recently, which meant she needed me gone, so she could prove herself to her bosses. My first day back, she gave me impossible goals and tasks to achieve, obviously designed for me to fail and justify her getting rid of me. Life took a drastic downturn. I was hit with overwhelming despair and fear. What would I do? We had no family or anywhere to go. She stripped me of my title and put me at a lower level position. I cannot describe to you the hell I plunged into that day. The panic, anxiety, and despair hit like I had never felt before in my life. My wife and kids were still in Brazil, so I had to endure this alone. I suffered. Oh, how I suffered. My mind went to the worst place possible, and suddenly there was no hope in sight. I tried to stay focused and on task, but nothing helped. In my mind, life was over, and my wife and children would be better off if I were gone. They could stay in Brazil with family and survive. I had nothing more to offer them. My world was destroyed.

Remarkably, during this time, I actually managed not only to meet the unattainable, unheard-of goals my boss had given me, but I surpassed them. I hoped this would make everything better, especially since she still had to rely on me to run the division, since she didn't know what she was doing. I managed not only to improve business but to save the company tens of thousands of dollars in losses. But this just seemed to make her more determined. She took away my assistant, which forced me to work even longer hours, and tried to find any way she could to strip more and more away and force me to leave. But I needed this job to provide for my family. After about nine months of utter hell, she came in with her boss and told me to leave. They had decided I was violating some rule or something and terminated my employment. I had lost my job, and soon we would lose our home. We had nothing. I couldn't believe they were willing to destroy a family for their own vain ambition. I was angry.

It was funny, though, because initially it was a bit of relief that the torture, she was putting me through was finally over. But what would I do now? Not only did I lose my job, but we lost our apartment and were homeless. We found a place to stay in another state, which was depressing enough, but we knew our time there would be limited. I am grateful for the charity my family received there, but we knew it wouldn't last, and eventually we were asked to leave. During this time, I kept having reoccurring dreams that I couldn't stand because my legs were not strong enough to support me. I felt so helpless and useless. I searched and searched for work. I found a job in Calgary, which was a good opportunity, so we went up to Canada to try to find housing and get documentation for my wife and kids, but nothing was working out, and eventually we were forced to come back to the States. My depression, anxiety, and suffering just intensified from there. Finally, after thirteen months of being homeless and jobless, an opportunity opened up, and I jumped at it. I was optimistic that things would finally be OK. We moved states again, and I started in my new job. It was with a good company that I had worked with in the past, and I hoped for a bright future.

My job was a new role for the company, however, and it would take time to build. This was not very good for someone who had been dealing with so much rejection, depression, and anxiety. Even now that I had a new job, money was still tight, and life was hard. Every day, I worried and feared I would lose my job and be out on the street again. All I ever wanted for my wife and kids was to give them a life I never had, one of stability and growth, but it seemed like we kept losing everything, including hope for the future. Year after year passed, but the depression and anxiety did not go away. In fact, it kept intensifying. I had lost what little self-confidence I had and just couldn't, for as hard as I tried, get better and just be OK. I could not find peace of mind. It was torture. Time after time, I fought the powerful thoughts of suicide. In my mind it seemed like the only option. I justified it by thinking my family would be so much better off without me. I saw myself as the screw up who caused all this heartache and suffering.

It was a battle each and every day to find a reason to carry on. Somehow, I did, though. I needed to, for the sake of my family.

CHAPTER 2

Trying to See in The Dark – Living with Anxiety and Depression

Now that you have the background of what brought me into the worst depression and anxiety I would ever feel, this chapter will discuss the challenges of day to day life living with depression and anxiety.

When the depression and anxiety hit the hardest, I was lost and unsure what to do. I also felt like I had no resources and was on my own. The lack of security, or hope for the future, of course, led me to even greater depression and anxiety. One of the biggest challenges with dealing with these two conditions is the stigma associated with it. Those who suffer aren't crazy, stupid, or weak. The world doesn't see illness of the mind the same way they see illness of the body, which is strange when you consider how studies have shown that when someone is in a good mental state, their body heals faster and stronger than if they are in a poor state of mind.

To put things in the simplest terms possible, trying to function each day with depression and anxiety is pure torture. There just seems to be no hope in the world. No reason to carry on.

Even though I had found a good job and a place to live, and even though that all seemed great, I was still very insecure and lost. I felt like I was going to lose my job at any moment, and we would be worse off than before. My mind would not allow me to feel secure. I lived in constant fear, overthinking every situation and taking every interaction negatively and very personally. I couldn't see any joy in life and couldn't see a future. Every day was one torturous event after another. If something would go right, I was sure it wouldn't last because something even worse was waiting just around the corner to destroy it and my peace. When my depression was at its worst, I often strongly contemplated suicide. I had to end it. I just couldn't handle any more of this suffering. I was in agony and life wasn't worth living. What was the point of going on? I have to admit, if it weren't for my wife and kids, I would have ended it many years ago.

I managed to find a therapist, and she was shocked to hear what I was going through mentally and emotionally. After a few sessions, she diagnosed me with Post-Traumatic Stress Disorder (PTSD) and tried many techniques to help me. One of her efforts included hurting me even more, emotionally, with the idea that my brain would flip into a defensive mode and fight back or something, to start healing or have a positive reaction. Sadly, it didn't produce the desired results, and she just made me feel worse. After each visit I was even closer to committing suicide. After a couple more sessions, during which I felt like I was losing my mind, she told me I was beyond her help and needed to find another therapist.

She referred me to a couple people and eventually I found one I liked. This therapist was better, but after she confirmed the diagnoses of PTSD, she determined that I needed to be medicated. I didn't disagree, because I was suffering so badly. I was desperate to find a solution and way to feel better. Each day was a struggle to get out of bed and face the world. The only thing that truly kept me going was my family. They needed me, and if I failed, how would they survive? I wanted to run away. I wanted so badly to escape this life and world. Oh, how I suffered. It was indescribable. I would never wish this kind of despair and pain upon my worst enemy. It was terrible. I apologize if I keep repeating myself at this point about how bad it was, but it is very hard to clearly describe the despair, fear, anxiety, and depression I went through. But I expect if you are reading this, you know what I am talking about. The world becomes so very dark and depressing.

So, I began the game of finding the right medication. One after another was tried, at different dosages, and nothing was ever really effective. Finally, I found the best one, that if taken in high dosages made life somewhat bearable. My senses seemed dulled, making life a little easier, but I still felt the depression and anxiety. They were still there, destroying my peace and leaving me with little hope. I just couldn't get past it. Along with the depression and anxiety, I now had physical issues. I felt ill all the time. Life was not worth living. I would go out each day hoping someone would run a red light and take me out, or someone would rob a store I was in and shoot me dead. I kept imagining and hoping for ways to die. I just couldn't keep going. I needed out. What is the point of living like this? My whole life had been a struggle and filled with suffering, pain and disappointment. What was the point of keeping that going?

Once again, if not for my family, I would have gotten off this terrible ride a long time ago. I realized that as terrible as things felt to me, I just couldn't do that to them. They were just starting in life; did they really need the trauma of their father dying? If I did die, what hope would they have for a stable future? I loved them too much to do that to them. So, I kept going, as hard as it was, year after year, suffering. After less than one year, I could no longer afford to see the therapist and was forced to go it alone again. The withdrawal from the medications I was on was terrible. I was sick for a long time, and as the medication left my system, the depression and anxiety were that much stronger. What was I to do?

Year after year the torture continued. It seemed like there was no hope. But I couldn't give up. I just couldn't, for the sake of my family. I had to keep fighting and trying to find a way out. And so, I started my journey to find better mental health.

CHAPTER 3

The Journey of Discovery – Finding Solutions to Overcome Anxiety and Depression

I am not going to tell you there is a miracle cure or method that will change your life. I am also not going to claim that what works for me will work for you. What I am going to tell you is there are things you can do that will help you overcome anxiety and depression and even find peace. Finding the right thing or things will be your key to success. It may take some experimentation, but you should keep fighting and looking for what helps you the most. Search for what is going to get you where you need to be mentally and emotionally. In this chapter I will describe some options that I have found to be the most beneficial for me, that brought me the greatest potential for relief from the suffering. I am sharing these things because I know they are not exclusive to me and could help anyone who is trying to find relief.

The key is having an open mind when it comes to finding the right methods and approaches that will help you. But the truth is, if you truly do suffer as I have, you are at the point in your life where you are willing to try anything to get the relief you need. Yet, even if you aren't a sufferer of severe anxiety or deep depression, there are a lot of things you can do to help yourself combat negative feelings and feel happier.

There are many causes or triggers of depression and anxiety

in this world. Try to identify the causes or triggers in your life that cause you to go down the negative path that leads to anxiety and depression. If you have a leaking pipe, you cannot fix it until you turn off the source of the water first. Once that is off, you can seal the hole causing the water to leak out. For some of us there are many holes in the pipe that need to be fixed, so it may take some time to identify all of them. According to the World Health Organization some commits suicide every 40 seconds around the world. That is over 800,000 suicides annually, and yet, healthcare for mental health is surprisingly lacking.

Next, try to find your motivation to keep going each day. That is one important key to finding peace. Find your reason to wake up each day, get out of bed, go out in the world, work, fight, and carry on, no matter how much it hurts. If you don't find your reason, you are going to struggle more. But each of you has a reason to keep going. I know in your mind you think you are alone, and nobody cares about you, but that is not true. Do not convince yourself that you are not important to those around you, be it family, friends, whatever. It is worth it to keep fighting and keep going. YOU have a lot to offer the world! You have many talents and abilities that need to be shared with everyone around you.

For me, my motivation to keep going was my family. My wife and kids. They were all I had in this world. The irony in my mind was that they were all I cared about and loved and kept me going, yet it was because of my need to provide for them that I was feeling this way. I felt like a failure to my family, but they were the reason I couldn't give up. I know they needed me to be strong. What is important to you? I have found that everyone has something they treasure or desire in life that will keep them going. Find or identify what yours is and focus on that each day.

The next method that I found to be one of the most effective for me was journal-writing. Journal-writing is the greatest therapist I can think of. How often have you had a question or concern and asked or started talking to someone about it, and before the other person even responds, you've figured out the answer? The act of just putting things into words can make a big difference in your thoughts and patterns. Journal-writing is an excellent way to do that. How you do it is your choice. I use a computer and prefer to type out my thoughts and feelings. I do it as often as needed, but I find I write more when I am feeling low, depressed, or anxious about something. Since I discovered journal-writing, I have written over 1600 pages totaling over 1.3 million words. Some of my writing is crazy and dark, and some is light and inspiring. But the point is to get your thoughts and feelings out on paper so you can see them from outside of your head. I cannot tell you how many times I have talked myself off a ledge just by expressing my feelings on paper or on a computer screen.

When you take time to write out your thoughts and feelings, it allows you to validate them or even dismiss them. It helps you take a closer look at what you are thinking or feeling and react more constructively. Do your feelings have merit? Are the negative thoughts you are experiencing warranted? I have found that most people who experience anxiety and depression are classic overthinkers like me. Oh man, do I overthink things. But when I write in my journal it really helps me stop overthinking. Write it out. Write it all out, then read and ponder what you wrote so you can start to let it go. It helps you move on and stop focusing on that same thought or idea that may be dragging you down.

Once you write out your thoughts and feelings, you can look back at them and often realize how out of touch they are. We fear and worry about so much. It is hard to escape those negative thoughts and feelings, especially when we don't take the time to look at the sources and causes – the holes in the pipe. Writing out things can help you do that. It helps you see things from the perspective of a third party and will give you an opportunity to see what is wrong and think of ways you can fix it.

I identified my triggers and found motivation to carry on, and the journal writing helped me think clearer. It all led me to look for solutions to finally overcome the anxiety and depression and everything that made me lose hope. Because of how bad it was, I knew I needed professional help. My next step was finding a mental health professional that could help me navigate the murky waters of my damaged mind. As I explained earlier, finding the right therapist was not an easy process. I went through a few therapists before finding one I felt like I was making progress with, but that progress was primarily through chemical assistance. Just going through the process of finding a medication that would help me brought me hope that I might be OK, though. It was a slow process to find one that helped at all. I was in such bad shape that I was actually researching how to get a lobotomy. I wanted to just cut out the part of my brain that made me care or even think. I thought it would be better to be unfeeling than to suffer day after day.

Now the truth is, I didn't find any medication to be very helpful, but what I did find was that one did help enough to let me think more clearly. That allowed me to begin looking for other methods of combating the effects of depression and anxiety. Personally, I don't think medications are the best answer, but this is my belief and it may work out differently for you. For me, to truly overcome depression and anxiety, medications were just a band-aid and becoming dependent on them would not have helped me in the long term. Again, I am not opposed to chemical or professional help; it did help me. But the true success I have found has been from things I have done on my own, rather than any help from medicine or a professional therapist.

As I mentioned earlier, I have found some help with medication, and maybe it is very effective for some; but for me, it was just a numbing cream to not feel my feelings. But they never really went away. It's probably the same effect as turning to alcohol or drugs to "escape" reality. I really don't blame anyone for doing that; when you are hurting and suffering, you just want it to stop. You do whatever you can to forget or stop the feelings from getting worse. The constant torture and suffering are also what leads so many to suicide. The pain can get so unbearable at times it seems like the only option. I have been there, I have suffered, and I have wished for death on many occasions. It pains me to think that others are going through that as well. One of my goals for writing this book is to help you or someone you know find ways to overcome the pain and discover how you can finally experience the peace you seek. There is too much suffering in this world. I know it is possible to combat this suffering if we fight for ourselves and others who suffer.

Let's return to trying to find out what causes emotional pain and suffering. Where we spend our time and focus will determine our outcome. What do you read, watch, study, and focus your time on throughout the day? Some of the worst places to spend your mental energy are on things like social media and the news. Not to say they don't offer positive things, but there are a lot of negative things out there that can bring you down mentally and emotionally, exposing you to greater chances at feeling depression and anxiety. For example, one email I got today read, "What to do if you feel like you are going to lose your job." For some, this might be a good proactive approach to getting ahead of the issue. But for me, the article had no real substance and could only lead me down the path of greater worry, thus triggering my anxiety or depression because I would start thinking that I may be at risk of losing my job again. But I know this is a trigger for me: the fact of the matter is, if I spend all my time worrying about losing my job, I tend to be much less effective than if I didn't have those thoughts. I had a co-worker who also struggled with this. Every time the boss's door would shut, she worried that it was about her and she would lose her job any day. This obsession led to inaction and failing to do her work, and, in the end, she did end up losing her job.

One of the challenges we face when dealing with anxiety and depression is that it zaps the desire and energy to act. It puts those who suffer into a state of inactivity and even fear of action, which leads to the moments when you just don't want to get out of bed. We seek peace, and a safe place where we don't have to face the trials of life that lie before us. After I lost my job and we were homeless, I found I was dwelling on social media, seeing what all my friends were doing and feeling left out and alone. I knew I had to cut off my social media if I was going to be okay. So that was one of the first things I did.

What gets us in that depressed or anxious state depends on the individual and whatever their triggers are. I bring up social media because it is one of mine: it is a world where everyone you know seems to be perpetually on vacation and having a good time with all their friends except for you. Following people who aren't truly your friends can lead you into a false sense of reality. Technology has made negative influences easier to find and dwell on. From the safety of our homes we can easily participate in extreme discussions regarding politics, religion, race, etc. These are not positive influences and can easily bring you down, leaving you with deep anxiety and depression. We must accept that many other people do not share our thoughts, feelings and opinions. If we allow others to dominate our thinking, we will never be truly happy.

The news is another source of negativity. I will use my father as an example on this one. The only thing he would watch on TV was the news and based on the coverage of negative events in the world, my father's view on life and the world was very bleak indeed. When I was just getting done with high school and looking to start life, if I sat and listened to my father make statements like, "The world is over. It's a disaster and there is no point with going on and living because of the government this and that, and robbers, muggers, murders, etc.", I wouldn't have been able to live a happy existence. Seeing his view on life and the world, as taught to him by the news, has taught me that there is little to no value in watching the news. Instead of watching the news, focus on the good in the world. There are plenty of positive programs and things you can watch and see that can help you restore your faith in the world and humanity.

What we focus on will determine our attitude about life and the amount of anxiety and depression we may experience. We really do live in an amazing world filled with wonderful things to see, do, and experience. But on the flipside, we are also surrounded by the negative aspects of this world that will attack and hurt you if you allow them to. As easily as technology can take you around the world and let you experience wonderous things, it can also be the cause of a lot of pain and suffering. The internet, social media, apps, and games offer great escapes, but if you aren't careful, you can get consumed by them and find yourself in a desperate place. I am a bit of a geek and love to build computers and play video games. There was a time that I would spend every waking moment immersed in online gaming, to the point of losing myself. But, like alcohol or drugs, they just don't do anything good in the long term for you. They are just quick fixes that you typically end up paying for later. The goal is learning to overcome the challenges of depression and anxiety long term, so you don't have to turn to unsafe and other harmful substances for relief.

It is very important that you identify all the sources of negative influences in your life. Then determine what can you do to change them. Sometimes, negative influences come from family or friends. Toxic relationships are never good for anyone. I will rarely encourage you to end family relationships. You should work hard to maintain strong families because, in the end, they may be all you have. However, there are some instances where the relationship is abusive, and that is not what a family should be. You need to remove yourself from abusive relationships as soon as possible. Those tend to lead to worse things than anxiety and depression. Choose your friends wisely. Do they make you a better person? Do you feel better about yourself when you are around them? If not, find friends that build you up and support you instead of breaking you down and making you feel worthless. This world is filled with wonderful people, and you can find them.

It has been said that happiness and contentment are a

choice. I have pondered this idea a lot and, as hard as it is to accept, I have come to the conclusion that it is true. But before you say, "How insulting. Do you really think I can simply *choose* not to be depressed or feel anxiety? Do you really think I can *choose* to just be fine?" No, I don't believe that. Believe me, I have tried. This statement is not about saying to yourself, "I am happy and okay, and I choose not to feel depressed or anxious," then suddenly you are happy. What it is saying is that you can find ways to overcome depression and anxiety by the choices you make each day. For instance, if you feel depressed by your weight or how you look, choose to change your eating habits and add exercise to your day. Making daily choices that have a direct impact on what is causing the anxiety or depression you feel is how you choose to be happy. In cases of more serious depression and anxiety like I have experienced, I came to a point where I just didn't want to suffer anymore. I was desperate to be better and function normally. So, the first choice I made in my quest to be happy was to seek professional help. Being able to discuss my issues in an open and safe place was very helpful. Even the process of finding the right medication and dosage was helpful, because it helped me see some light at the end of the tunnel. Just making the choice to find a solution begins the path to overcoming the depression and anxiety that drain you every day.

This is a critical time because maybe you have learned to function with anxiety and depression, or maybe not, but one day you will be tired, worn out, and might feel like you just can't keep going that way anymore. I plead for you to act now to make changes in your life before you get to a point when you are willing to hurt yourself. I understand how much it hurts and how bad you feel -- like you are in quicksand or a muddy pit, and no matter how much you try, you seem to just keep sinking deeper and deeper, and you are just so tired you can't find the strength to keep going. But don't stop. Don't give up. There is hope, and there is help. I don't care who you are, you have people who love you and want to help you. Find them and let them help you.

CHAPTER 4

The Results – What I Found Most Helpful

After a lot of trial and error, I found there are a few things that help me, find success. This chapter is a truer chronological order of my approach to overcoming anxiety and depression, in which I will discuss each of the methods I have used and how much I believe they have helped my progress. I am not trying to tell you or anyone that this is the best or only approach. I am six foot nine inches tall; I know all too well that one size does not fit all. My goal here is to offer a few techniques that can help. I hope you will experiment with the different techniques and find the key to overcoming your anxiety and depression, so you can finally enjoy some peace and happiness.

I truly believe the world we live in is all in our mind. How you see life, and your experiences of your day to day life, will impact how you think and feel. We all know those individuals who are negative about everyone and everything they see. We also know those people who always seem so happy. Your perspective on life will impact your overall well-being. You can take two different people and put them through the same experience, and each will have a different reaction. The one in a good mental state will have enjoyed or at least learned from the experience while the other, in a poor mental state, will say it was boring or terrible or even painful. How we mentally approach life will ultimately determine the results -- the life we live being filled with suffering and pain, or joy and happiness. The best example I can give for this is from the year we took the kids to South America to visit family. Mind you, we were traveling from North America to a developing country where we wouldn't be staying in fancy hotels and in areas that they have all the modern conveniences we have here. It can be a bit of a culture shock when you first get there, and even though I have been many times, it takes some adjustment at first. Our oldest son was in his teen years and did not want to go. He complained the whole way there and grumbled for days. He was miserable for most of the trip while we all had a good time. After a period of time, though, he started to enjoy himself. Before he knew it, it was time for us to head home, and that is when he wished he could stay longer. If we fail to open our eyes to wonderful life experiences, it will be very hard to find happiness and peace.

As I previously mentioned, my first effort to find happiness and peace by overcoming my anxiety and depression was to try to understand what was causing my issues. What were my triggers that left me feeling depressed or anxious? This was very hard to do at first because overthinking situations made it very hard to pinpoint anything. From there, I changed gears by trying to focus my mind on better things. I tried to read books and spend my time on good, positive, uplifting things. I turned to religion and sought counsel and guidance, but the truth is, those whom I talked to didn't understand what I was going through and offered little help. The crazy thing was, I may have shown a calm demeanor, or at least appeared relatively calm on the outside, but inside I was screaming out in terrible pain, hoping someone, anyone could hear me and save me from this suffering. It was the worst pain and suffering I would ever experience, and I know I have already expressed this, but truthfully, I would never wish it on my worst enemy. It was excruciating torture. Unfortunately, this suffering would be my life for many years to come. Sure, I had brief moments of being at peace, but they were very short-lived.

I can't say that religion, therapy, and books didn't help me at all; they did help me find some focus and think more outside of myself, and this was an excellent stepping stone to get me on the right path. It was religion that most helped me look more outward, and what I saw were my kids and my wife and how much I loved them. I knew I had to find the strength to carry on for their sakes. I wondered where they would be without me. My wife had always been a stay-at-home mother and taken care of the kids and me. Even though my wife eventually went to college, got her degree, and is trying to start a career in teaching, I have always been the main provider for my family. I had to keep going so I could give them the future and a life I felt I never had. I was failing, but I just couldn't give up.

Focusing on them really helped me survive. Find something important to you. Find someone or something you love, that makes you want to keep fighting and live. Even though this didn't get me out of my depression and anxiety, it gave me reason to carry on. To keep fighting. This meant I kept getting up each morning and trying to do what needed to be done to provide for the family. When you have someone or something that depends on you, it's possible to find the motivation to keep going, even though it's hard, and it will be one of the best things you can do. As I look back and think about how often and how long I was suffering through anxiety and depression, it makes me feel bad to think how much I missed out on with my kids. I was physically present for big events in their lives, but I was never there mentally or emotionally, and that really hurts. Our family and friends really need us to be present in their lives. I recognized that if I wanted my kids to be more emotionally stable, I had to find a way to be there for them emotionally, too. My family was one of the strongest drivers for finding a way to get through my anxiety and depression. Even recognizing how important they were to me, this wasn't the cure, it was one of the biggest motivating factors for me to keep going and try everything I could to keep fighting. I saw a quote recently that said, "She's gonna forever say 'I got this,' even with tears in her eyes". It did not have an author, but I thought this spoke volumes about what we need to do to get through this and overcome this suffering we feel. The true key is never giving up! You are strong enough! Keep going, keep fighting! I promise you that there is always hope and you are worth it. You have great value to more people than you know. Never sell yourself short or let yourself believe that you are worthless or hopeless.

The next and probably one of the best techniques I tried was journal-writing. A few years ago, while I was preparing for a presentation, I was trying to think straight and figure out how to develop the talking points, and I remembered a technique I had used in the past called mind-mapping. This is a technique similar to brainstorming that allows you to just write out your thoughts in whatever direction they go. It can really help you think through what is going on in your brain. But this particular time, I found it really helped me focus my mind and think more clearly, by stepping outside my thoughts and looking at them in a more focused manner. This process really allowed me to think about my issues, anxieties, and depression, and the next thing I knew, my thoughts were out on paper. This was a remarkable day for me. For the first time, I felt like I was stepping outside of myself and looking at my problems in a whole new light. I was finally able to look at everything differently, talk myself down off the ledge and focus my mind more. One of the biggest problems with anxiety and depression is being stuck in a loop of negativity and dark thoughts. When you can write out your thoughts, it allows you to see them differently. You can then scrutinize your own thinking, and more times than not, you can see where your thinking is going wrong. It allows you to take a step back and reevaluate your thinking and clear your mind. Now, I am not saying this is a perfect process or even a quick fix, but I have talked myself down on many occasions. There have been times when I have written for hours at a time and spent most of that time writing in circles -- repeating my feelings and thoughts so I could validate them and then work through how they were either without foundation or understanding that they were merely fears and negative thoughts that just hurt and brought me down emotionally. This is never an easy or simple process no matter what method you use. But what I did find was that journal writing had the greatest long-term impact in my overall mental health.

Even using these first techniques of identifying my triggers, finding my motivation to keep going, and journal-writing, it still wasn't enough for me, and I knew I needed more help. I sought counseling and support. I didn't have much money, and counseling can be expensive, but luckily, I found help with paying for some sessions. A lot of companies today offer employee assistance programs that provide free counseling and other help. Sure, it's limited, but it could be the start you need, and then once you get going you can find programs that can help you carry on with counseling if needed.

In my case it was just what I needed. I had a rocky start, though, as the first counselor used an approach and theory where they try and call your feelings out in an aggressive manner. I believe the theory behind this is to get you to fight and overcome those feelings, like the idea that if you are afraid of heights, then you should go stand on the tallest buildings and other high places in order to overcome your fears. This method did not help me at all. Quite frankly, it sent me into a downward spiral, and I was closer to committing suicide after each session. I told the therapist to stop during one session, and she tried to understand why it wasn't working; but, in the end, she suggested another therapist because she didn't know how to help me. I was in a very dark place and she was making me worse. But just like with doctors trying to find the right treatment to fix your ailing or broken body, everyone is different. Even though this method did not work for me, it may work for you. I recommend you keep an open mind and keep trying till you find what does work.

The first therapist quickly diagnosed me with severe PTSD and gave me the card of another therapist. I scheduled an appointment with the new therapist and found a more comforting situation. After a couple sessions she decided I really needed chemical assistance in order to get through this, so we began the process of finding the right concoctions that would help me. It took a while and the dosages where quite high until we found what seemed to work best. Some people need medication for anxiety and depression for the rest of their lives, but I knew this would not be a long-term fix for me, personally. I just didn't want to rely on drugs to maintain my sanity. The medicine did help me think clearer and help me focus more, though, and with it I could continue looking for solutions to get better and overcome the crippling effects of anxiety and depression.

It took quite a few months, but after we found the right medications that worked best for me, I could finally function better. Was this a cure? Not at all. I still felt the anxiety and depression, and still had moments of panic and hard times, but it helped give me the power to make it more manageable for me. If the first techniques I listed are not enough for you, or if it is very hard for you to deal with life, please find professional help and, if recommended by your therapist or doctor, get on some medication so you can function well enough to find a long-term solution that works for you.

The next technique I implemented to help myself was meditation. There are all kinds of meditation apps and videos that you can use for free. The advantage of meditation is that it helps focus your thoughts on more productive areas. The simple act of finding a calm, quiet place and focusing on your breathing is amazingly powerful. Truth be told, I thought meditation was garbage and could never work for me. So, at first, I didn't believe I could benefit from this process, because quiet places are where my mind would go crazy and I would circle the drain. But when you learn to focus your thoughts and mind, you can find yourself in a more peaceful state. I find that listening to stories helps me a lot because it focuses my mind on that rather than the negativity that keeps coming back to my mind. But there are many meditation options out there you can try.

These were the things that finally got me on the path to

finding a more lasting solution to overcoming anxiety and depression. I found myself coming full circle on these techniques and using all of them at once, but at this point, the one I started focusing on more was religion. Whether you believe in God or not, there are a lot of beliefs and practices along the same vein that can help you find peace. The feelings of anxiety and depression trap us within ourselves, so finding a way to get out of your own head and focusing on others can be a real benefit. What I mean by this is service to and helping others. When we can focus on others, we can step outside of ourselves and find greater satisfaction and peace. I know this sounds crazy; I can imagine you asking, "How in the world can I help others and serve others when I can't even help myself?" But it's true, you can. Yes, it's hard, especially at first. But as you keep trying, it gets easier and easier, and you can find yourself in a great place emotionally the more you do it. This is what I did. Truth is, as hard of a time as I was having, I was amazed to find how many other people are struggling with this or other serious issues themselves. I have yet to meet someone who couldn't use a friendly smile, a hug, or a simple *how are you doing today*. Seek to serve and help others and you will find how small your problems truly are.

One of the things I found that kept me in a deep depression was comparing myself with others. But the truth is, I was comparing myself with what I perceived, what I thought others were like. In my mind, everything had worked out perfectly for everyone around me. Too often, we fool ourselves into thinking everyone else is doing great and we are the only ones struggling with life's challenges, and that is a dangerous path to take. It is a deep, dark hole that will swallow us up if we allow it to. This is why I have cautioned against social media. It is a trap that can make you believe everyone has the perfect life except you. One of the healthiest things I did was turn off all my social media accounts. I have since turned a couple back on, but I am very selective of who and what I follow and look at. I don't care about how many friends I have; I focus on following inspiring organizations and people who lift me up and help me feel better about myself and life. Purge the life-draining negativity from your world. There is so much good out there that you can feed on instead to help strengthen and fortify you.

In addition, I found many YouTube videos that are helpful and uplifting. A couple are called Fear, and I watched them about a million times, as they are very motivating. I also follow a few boards on Pinterest that offer wonderful quotes and ideas that help me when I am feeling down. Look for the good and focus on what helps you the most. The world has wonderful people and things to help you. Many others are struggling with challenges of their own. You are not alone.

CHAPTER 5

The Future

Have I got it all figured out? Certainly not. This life is a journey and I believe we are here for a greater purpose. Our goal should be finding a way to be better today than we were yesterday. Overcoming anxiety and depression and finding peace and happiness is not a sprint; it is a marathon. Good mental health is just like trying to lose weight: it is a lifestyle change and an ongoing process, even after you reach your goals. Along the way you will find the tools and techniques that will allow you to be better. You will have good days and bad days. I have had days and weeks that were very good, and I have had weeks and months that were very bad. But what we all need to do is learn from each experience and find what works best and use it. An idea I like to focus on and that I use a lot is that *I didn't come this far just to come this far*. Keep fighting and you will find the peace and relief from anxiety and depression one day. It doesn't come all at one time, but piece by piece. Just like in school, we learn little by little and build upon concepts until we have a greater understanding. Overcoming anxiety and depression is the same.

No two of us are the identical, though, so what works for me may not work for you. But what I am hoping to share here is that you can find what works for you if you fight for it. I got tired of the constant suffering. I just couldn't live like that anymore, because I was going to break. The mind can only take so much, and if I didn't find a solution, I would have made the worst possible decision: to end my life. Don't let yourself get there. Too many people think there is no hope and seeing statistics for suicides in this world is shocking. It makes me sad to see so many people suffering as I have. It makes me sad that they got to the point of thinking they couldn't take it anymore and life wasn't worth living. The impact of such a decision has lasting effects, and I don't just mean for you. It has huge impacts on your family and friends as well. I beg anyone who is struggling with suicidal thoughts to find someone to they can talk to and find help to get out of that thought process.

I hate to say it, but I did not find the suicide hotline that I called helpful at all. I felt like they were just trying to push me off on emergency services. It may be different in other places, but I wish the one I called would have understood that if someone is calling, what they really need is someone to talk to. A friendly voice who cares and offers support could be all they need. Often, people just need someone to listen with a sympathetic ear and help talk them down. I understand that suicide hotlines can be overburdened and might not have the manpower or resources or time to sit and talk to someone, but that could be the difference between life and death. What really makes me sad is the lack of resources and support for those suffering with mental health issues. We are largely left on our own unless we seek out help. Unless you come from a very wealthy family, you may think you have few options. But they are out there.

By this point, I wonder if you are curious to ask if I am free from anxiety and depression. A quick answer to that question is no, I am not free from these conditions, but I have learned how to better manage them and what techniques work the best for me when I am starting to feel down or anxious. I always try to break the pattern quickly, to avoid falling down that dark pit of despair.

No, I am not "cured," but I am headed in the right direction. I mentioned previously that I didn't want to become dependent on medications in order to maintain my mood or control my thoughts, and I haven't. But the medications helped me on the path to helping myself. After a time, I decided to wean myself off the medications and practice the things that help me stay centered. It has been hard, but I have been off the medications for almost two years now, and I am ok without them. Sure, there are bad days, but I now have ways to help me overcome them. Create a toolbox for yourself of techniques that help you. Although I think medications can be very helpful, at the end of the day you need to find ways to deal with your anxiety and depression -- to overcome them instead of just masking your feelings. Think before using alcohol, marijuana, or anything else that numbs your mind. It might feel like a good short-term fix, but once it wears off, you will be back to where you started -- and often in a worse place than where you started. Learn to control your feelings instead. Learn techniques that will empower you! Don't empower things that remove your free will by altering your consciousness with chemicals.

My goal in writing this book has been to help you understand that there is hope. Be open to new possibilities. Be open to new techniques. You can find ways to deal with crippling depression and anxiety and find the peace you never thought was possible. I believe we live on after this life and what we make of ourselves here will determine how we live beyond this life. You have the power within you to be stronger and overcome the mental and emotional challenges you face. You have more family and friends willing to help than you realize. Ask for help. Do not suffer in silence. Reach out and be willing to open up and get this out there. The more you share, the easier it is to overcome. Sure, there are those who will scoff and try and diminish your feelings, but don't let those ignorant people stop you. Keep fighting until you find the key to your peace and happiness. It is out there, and you can find it.

I know you are Wounded, but you have the power to be whole once again! Find the motivation to get up and fight for what you deserve! You deserve to be at peace and find true lasting happiness! Believe in yourself and your power to overcome the pain and suffering associated with anxiety and depression. There are those who love and depend on you. You are not alone!